Efficient

Fitness

Quick, Fast, and Easy Methods for Busy Professionals

FITGAL

Contents

Introduction

Welcome to Efficient Fitness: Quick, Fast, and Easy Methods for Busy Professionals!

Hi, I'm Fit Gal, and I'm thrilled to share with you some life-changing fitness strategies tailored specifically for busy professionals. In this guide, you will learn how to seamlessly integrate effective workouts into your daily routine, no matter how packed your schedule might be. We'll explore quick and efficient exercises, motivational tips, flexible fitness plans, and easy meal prep ideas that ensure you stay on track without feeling overwhelmed.

My Story

Years ago, I was exactly where you are now—juggling a demanding career, personal commitments, and a deep desire to stay fit and healthy. My days were filled with meetings, deadlines, and family responsibilities, leaving little time for myself. The thought of fitting in regular workouts seemed impossible, and I constantly battled with fatigue and stress.

One day, after another exhausting week, I had an epiphany. I realized that the key to maintaining fitness wasn't about finding more time; it was about making the most of the time I already had. I began to experiment with short, high-intensity workouts, simple meal preps, and practical routines that fit into my hectic schedule. The results were astounding—not only did I start feeling more energetic and focused, but I also saw significant improvements in my fitness levels.

The Secret Revealed

Here's the secret: You don't need hours at the gym to stay fit. By incorporating High-Intensity Interval Training (HIIT) and quick, effective exercises into your daily routine, you can achieve remarkable results in just 20 minutes a day. This approach not only saves time but also boosts your metabolism, burns more calories, and enhances your overall fitness. Imagine squeezing in a powerful workout during your lunch break or while dinner is cooking—yes, it's that easy!

What You Will Learn

1. **Efficient Workouts**: Discover the power of HIIT and other quick workout routines that can be done anywhere, anytime.
2. **Motivational Strategies**: Learn how to set achievable goals, track your progress, and stay motivated even on the busiest days.

3. **Flexible Fitness Plans**: Find out how to adapt your fitness routine to fit your unpredictable schedule without compromising results.
4. **Practical Meal Prep**: Get tips on preparing balanced, nutritious meals that save time and keep you energized throughout the week.
5. **Sustainable Habits**: Develop habits that integrate seamlessly into your daily life, making fitness a natural and enjoyable part of your routine.

Trust me, if I could transform my health and fitness amidst a chaotic lifestyle, so can you. Let's embark on this journey together and unlock your full potential with practical, efficient, and sustainable fitness solutions.

Chapter 1: Overcoming Time Constraints

Feeling like you can't squeeze in a workout? Trust me, I get it. But what if I told you that 20 minutes is all you need to stay fit? Let me introduce you to High-Intensity Interval Training (HIIT). This method combines short bursts of intense activity with brief rest periods. It fits perfectly into a packed schedule and maximizes calorie burn while boosting cardiovascular health. Imagine transforming a small part of your day into a powerhouse of fitness!

The Challenge: You and I both know how tough it is to balance a demanding schedule with fitness goals. With work deadlines, family responsibilities, and social commitments, finding time for exercise often takes a back seat.

The Strategy: Embrace short, high-impact workouts designed to deliver maximum results in minimal time.

Key Stats and Insights:

- **Statista Insight:** A significant 50% of Americans aged 18-64 report that lack of time is a major barrier to regular exercise.
- **Expert Endorsement:** "HIIT is not just a time-saver; it's a life-changer. It allows busy

professionals to achieve their fitness goals without compromising their schedules." – Nathan Richardson, CEO of a leading fitness company.

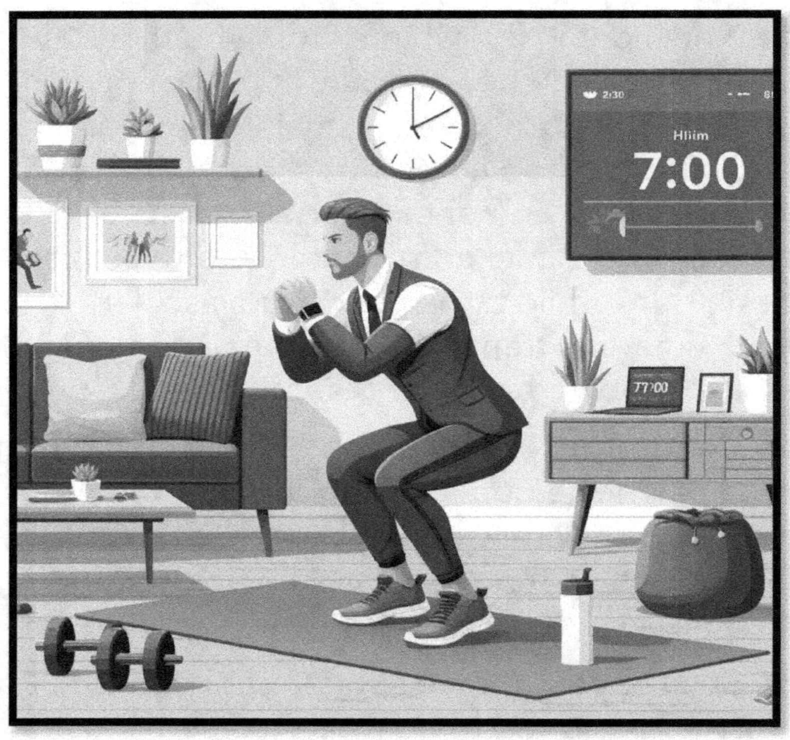

Quick HIIT workouts can fit into any busy schedule.

Paint a Picture:

Imagine this: It's 7:00 AM, and your day is already packed with meetings, projects, and errands. Instead of sacrificing your fitness goals, you spend just 20 minutes on a HIIT workout. You perform exercises like jump squats, burpees, and sprints in short, intense bursts, followed by brief rest periods. By 7:20 AM, you're done, energized, and ready to tackle your day. This efficient use of time means you've already checked off your workout before most people have finished their morning coffee.

Why It Works:

- **Efficiency:** HIIT workouts are designed to be completed in a short amount of time, making them ideal for busy schedules.
- **Effectiveness:** Research shows that HIIT can burn 25-30% more calories than other forms of exercise in the same amount of time.
- **Versatility:** HIIT can be performed anywhere—at home, in a park, or even in a hotel room during business trips.

Unique Example of a Morning HIIT Routine:

20-Minute Morning HIIT Routine for Busy Professionals:

1. Warm-Up (2 minutes):
   - Jumping Jacks: 1 minute
   - Arm Circles: 1 minute

2. Main Workout (16 minutes):
    o **High Knees:** 30 seconds
    o **Rest:** 15 seconds
    o Squat Jumps: 30 seconds
    o **Rest:** 15 seconds
    o Mountain Climbers: 30 seconds
    o **Rest:** 15 seconds
    o **Push-Ups:** 30 seconds
    o **Rest:** 15 seconds
    o **Burpees:** 30 seconds
    o **Rest:** 15 seconds
    o **Lunges:** 30 seconds
    o **Rest:** 15 seconds
    o **Plank:** 30 seconds
    o **Rest:** 15 seconds
    o **Repeat** the circuit 2 more times
3. Cool Down (2 minutes):
    o **Stretching:** Focus on major muscle groups (quads, hamstrings, shoulders, and back).

By rethinking how you approach fitness, you can integrate effective workouts into your daily routine without feeling overwhelmed. Embrace the power of HIIT and transform those precious 20 minutes into a gateway to better health and fitness.

Chapter 2: Finding and Sustaining Motivation

The Challenge: You're busy, I get it. With the whirlwind of work, family, and social obligations, staying motivated to exercise regularly can feel like an uphill battle. It's easy to start strong, but maintaining that drive is a different story.

The Strategy: Implement easy-to-follow fitness plans and adopt motivational strategies that keep you engaged and committed.

Let's Chat: Staying motivated to keep up with an exercise routine can be tough, especially when you're balancing so much. Here's a method that might help: set small, achievable goals and track your progress using fitness apps. Watching your improvements over time can be incredibly satisfying and keeps the motivation alive. Joining an online community or finding a workout buddy can also make a significant difference. When you have someone cheering you on and holding you accountable, it's easier to stay on track. Apps like MyFitnessPal or Strava provide social features that boost accountability and motivation.

Key Stats and Insights:

- **Statista Insight:** Approximately 35% of individuals who start a fitness program quit within the first six months due to lack of motivation.

- **Expert Quote:** "Motivation is what gets you started. Habit is what keeps you going." – Jim Ryun, former American track and field athlete.

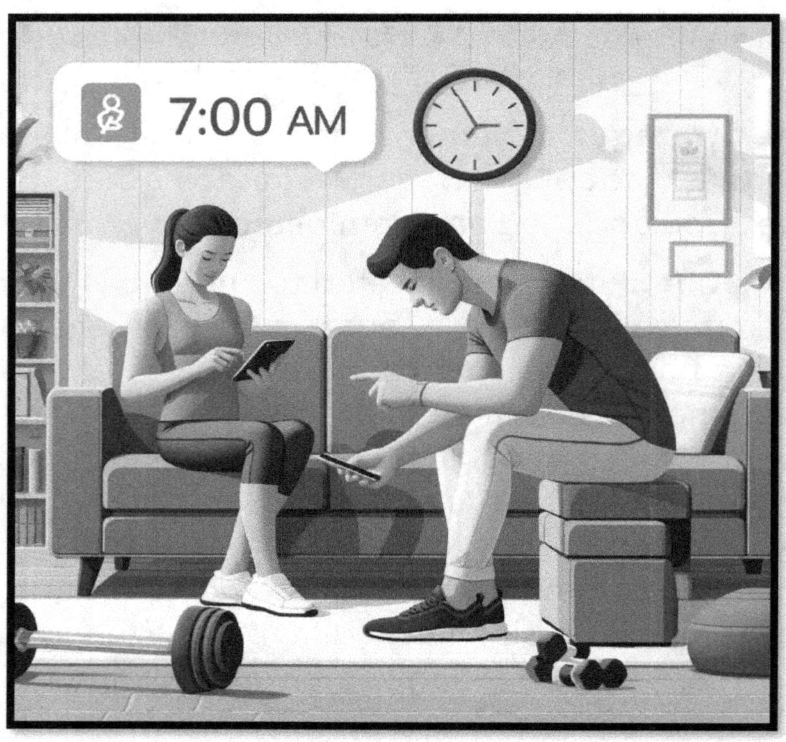

Fitness apps like MyFitnessPal can help track progress and keep you motivated.

Paint a Picture:

Imagine this: You've just wrapped up a long day at work, and the last thing you feel like doing is exercising. But you remember that you've set a goal to walk 10,000 steps a day. You open your MyFitnessPal app, see that you're only 2,000 steps away, and decide to take a brisk evening walk. As you walk, you feel your stress melting away, and you start to enjoy the fresh air. When you get back, you check your progress and see that you've not only met your goal but exceeded it. The satisfaction of seeing those numbers climb keeps you motivated to do it again the next day.

Why It Works:

- **Achievable Goals:** Setting small, realistic goals ensures that you can make steady progress without feeling overwhelmed.
- **Progress Tracking:** Using apps to log your activities helps you visualize your achievements, making it easier to stay motivated.
- **Community Support:** Engaging with online communities or finding workout buddies provides the encouragement and accountability you need to stick with your routine.

Featured Apps and Progress Tracking:

1. MyFitnessPal:
    - **Features:** Calorie counting, meal logging, and progress tracking. Screenshot:

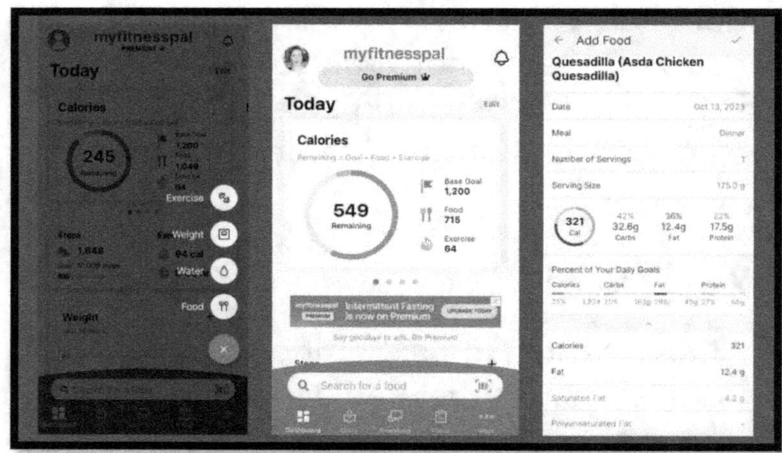

MyFitnessPal helps you stay on track with your fitness goals.

    - **Where to Find:** Available on the App Store and Google Play Store.
2. Strava:
    - **Features:** GPS tracking for running and cycling, social features to share progress.
    - Screenshot:

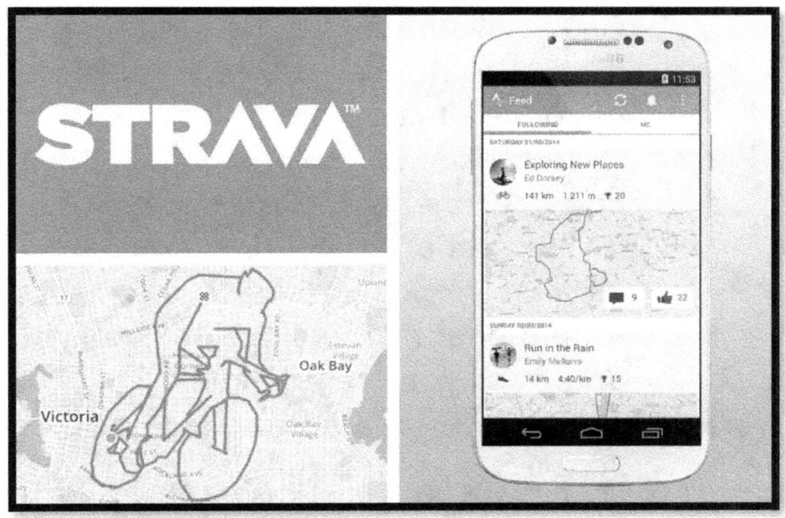

Strava's social features keep you motivated by connecting with friends and fellow athletes.

- o **Where to Find:** Available on the App Store and Google Play Store.

Specific Example of Implementing Easy-to-Follow Fitness Plans and Motivational Strategies:

Scenario: Busy Professional on the Go

What to Do:

1. Set a Realistic Goal:
   - o Open MyFitnessPal and set a goal to log 10,000 steps per day or track your daily calorie intake.
2. Plan Your Workouts:

- o Use Strava to map out a running or cycling route that you can complete in 30 minutes before or after work.

3. Track Your Progress:
   - o Log your meals and exercise in MyFitnessPal daily. For example, if you have a business trip, use the app to find healthy meal options nearby and track your calorie intake.
4. Stay Motivated with Community Support:
   - o Join a Strava club related to your interests or profession. Engage with other members by sharing your progress and participating in challenges.

Example Routine:

- **Morning:** Quick 10-minute HIIT session using a routine from a fitness app like Nike Training Club.
- **Lunchtime:** A brisk 15-minute walk, tracked on MyFitnessPal.
- **Evening:** A 20-minute run using a route mapped on Strava.

While Traveling:

- **Airport:** Use the airport terminal for brisk walking to hit your step goal.
- **Hotel:** Follow a bodyweight workout routine from MyFitnessPal or Strava.

- **Meals:** Log your food intake in MyFitnessPal to stay mindful of your nutrition.

Why It Works:

- **Flexibility:** These plans are adaptable to different environments, ensuring you can maintain your fitness routine regardless of location.
- **Accountability:** Tracking progress and engaging with a community keeps you motivated and accountable.
- **Convenience:** Using apps makes it easy to log activities and meals, providing a clear overview of your progress.

By focusing on setting achievable goals, tracking your progress, and engaging with supportive communities, you can maintain the motivation needed to integrate fitness into your daily life. Embrace these strategies and watch as they transform your fitness journey from a chore into a rewarding and sustainable part of your routine.

Chapter 3: Maintaining Consistency in a Busy World

The Challenge: You and I both know how hard it is to keep a consistent workout routine when your schedule is all over the place. Meetings pop up unexpectedly, deadlines shift, and personal commitments can disrupt even the best-laid plans. It feels like just when you get into a groove, something throws you off track.

The Strategy: Let's talk about flexible and adaptable fitness plans that can seamlessly fit into your daily life, no matter how chaotic things get. This approach helps you stay active even when you don't have a solid block of time to dedicate to exercise.

Let's Chat: I understand how unpredictable your schedule can be. That's why having a flexible workout plan is crucial. You can weave exercise into your daily routine through small, manageable activities. Think about doing desk exercises, taking walking meetings, or fitting in a quick workout during your lunch break. The goal is to make fitness a natural part of your day, ensuring you stay active regardless of your hectic schedule. For instance, you can do bodyweight exercises like squats and push-ups during short breaks.

Key Stats and Insights:

- **Statista Insight:** Over 60% of professionals report that inconsistent schedules make it challenging to maintain a regular fitness routine.
- **Expert Quote:** "Flexibility is key. You don't need a perfect routine, just a plan that works for you and adapts to your schedule." – Dean Lee, Head of Marketing at Sealions.

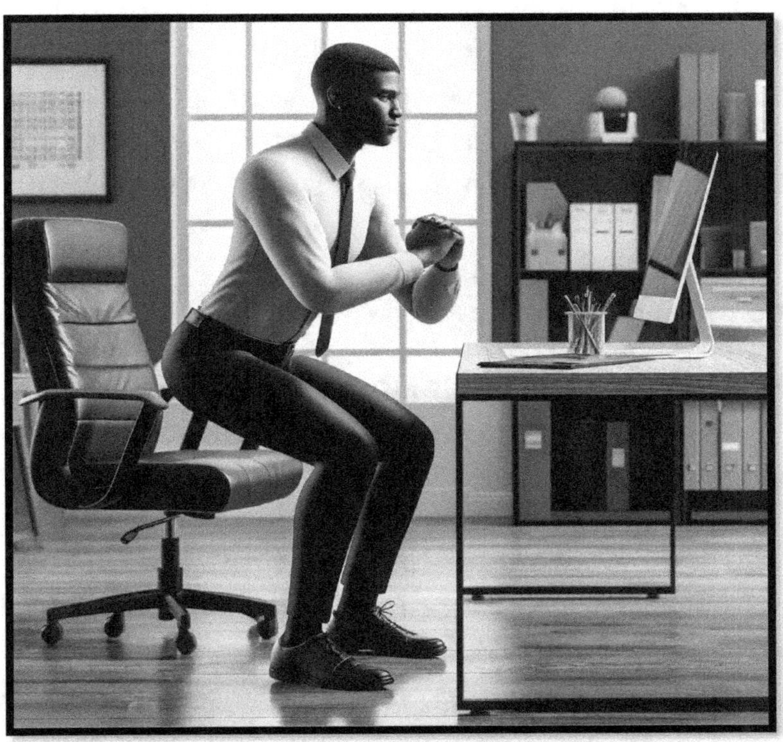

Desk exercises can help maintain consistency in your fitness routine.

Paint a Picture:

Imagine this: You're in the middle of a busy workday with back-to-back meetings. Finding time for a full workout seems impossible. But instead of skipping exercise altogether, you decide to incorporate movement into your routine. During a conference call, you stand up and do a few stretches and squats. Later, you take a walking meeting with a colleague, discussing business while you both get some fresh air and steps in. At lunch, you spend 10 minutes doing a quick bodyweight workout in your office or a quiet corner. By the end of the day, you've managed to stay active without needing to carve out a large block of time for the gym.

Why It Works:

- **Adaptability:** Flexible plans allow you to fit exercise into any part of your day, making it easier to stay consistent.
- **Integration:** By integrating small bouts of activity into your daily routine, you ensure that exercise becomes a natural and regular part of your life.
- **Efficiency:** Short, effective workouts can still provide significant health benefits,

helping you stay fit even when time is limited.

Specific Example of a Flexible Fitness Plan:

A Day in the Life of a Busy Professional:

1. Morning:
   - **Wake-Up Stretch (5 minutes):** Start your day with a quick stretch routine to wake up your muscles.
   - **Example:** Reach for the sky stretch, forward bends, and neck rolls.
2. Mid-Morning:
   - Desk Exercises (10 minutes):
     - **Exercises:** Chair squats, desk push-ups, and seated leg raises.
   - **Benefit:** These exercises can be done at your desk, ensuring you stay active even during work hours.
3. Lunch Break:
   - Quick Workout (15 minutes):
     - **Exercises:** Jumping jacks, lunges, and planks.
   - **Benefit:** A short, intense workout can boost your energy for the rest of the day.
4. Afternoon:
   - Walking Meeting (30 minutes):

- **Activity:** Discuss business matters while walking around your office building or a nearby park.
  - **Benefit:** Combines physical activity with work, maximizing productivity.

5. Evening:
   - Post-Dinner Walk (20 minutes):
     - **Activity:** A leisurely walk after dinner to aid digestion and relax.
   - **Benefit:** Helps you unwind and adds to your daily step count.

Tips to Stay Motivated and Reminded:

1. Set Reminders:
   - Use your phone or smartwatch to set reminders for your exercise breaks. Apps like MyFitnessPal and Strava have notification features that can remind you to stay active.
2. Visual Cues:
   - Place workout equipment like resistance bands or dumbbells in visible areas around your workspace to remind you to use them.
3. Goal Setting:
   - Set daily or weekly fitness goals. Track your progress using fitness

apps. Seeing your achievements can be a great motivator.

4. Social Accountability:
   - Share your fitness goals with friends or join an online fitness community. Social platforms within apps like Strava can help you stay accountable.
5. Rewards:
   - Treat yourself when you hit a fitness milestone. It could be something small like a favourite snack or a new workout outfit.
6. Incorporate Variety:
   - Change your workouts regularly to keep things interesting. Try different exercises or fitness classes to stay engaged.

By focusing on flexible and adaptable fitness plans, you can maintain consistency even with a busy schedule. Embrace these strategies and see how seamlessly fitness can fit into your life, turning exercise from a daunting task into a manageable and enjoyable part of your daily routine.

Chapter 4: Making Fitness Accessible Anywhere

The Challenge: You and I both know how tough it can be to stay fit without easy access to a gym or specialized fitness equipment. Whether it's due to the cost of memberships, the time it takes to get to the gym, or simply preferring to exercise at home, this lack of accessible resources can be a significant barrier.

The Strategy: Let's talk about how you can use home workouts and bodyweight exercises to stay fit. These methods require minimal to no equipment and can be incredibly effective.

Let's Chat: You don't need a gym to stay fit. There are plenty of effective workouts you can do right at home using just your body weight or simple equipment like resistance bands. Online workout programs and apps can guide you through these exercises, making it easy to stay fit without stepping out of your home. Imagine transforming your living room into a mini-gym where you can work out anytime! Resources like YouTube offer countless free workout videos that require no equipment.

Key Stats and Insights:

- **Statista Insight:** Home fitness equipment sales have surged by 170% during the COVID-19 pandemic, highlighting the shift towards home-based workouts.
- **Expert Quote:** "Your body is the best piece of equipment you own. Use it effectively, and you can achieve great results without ever stepping into a gym." – Tiffany Payne, Head of Content at PharmacyOnline.co.uk.

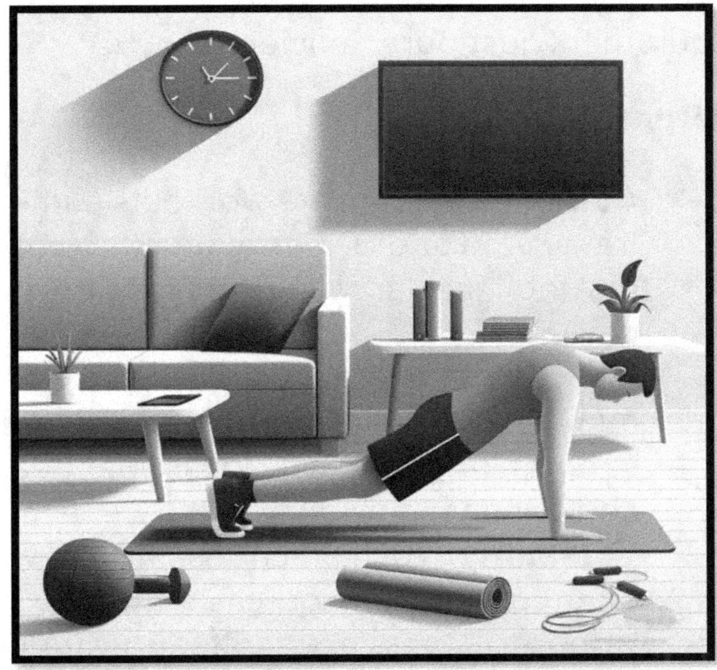

Effective home workouts require minimal equipment.

Paint a Picture:

Imagine this: It's early morning, and you're preparing to start your day. Instead of rushing to the gym, you roll out a yoga mat in your living room. With a quick glance at your phone, you open a workout app and follow a guided 20-minute HIIT session. You perform exercises like push-ups, squats, and burpees, all using just your body weight. The session is intense, yet satisfying. By the end of it, you're sweating and feeling accomplished, ready to tackle your workday. No commute, no waiting for equipment, just pure, efficient exercise.

Why It Works:

- **Convenience:** Home workouts eliminate travel time and gym membership costs, making it easier to fit exercise into your day.
- **Effectiveness:** Bodyweight exercises and minimal equipment workouts can build strength, improve cardiovascular health, and enhance flexibility.
- **Versatility:** You can choose from a wide range of online resources, from YouTube videos to fitness apps, offering various routines to keep things interesting.

Specific Example of a Home Workout Plan:

A Week of Home Workouts:

1. Monday: Full-Body Strength (30 minutes)
   - **Warm-Up (5 minutes):** Jumping jacks, high knees, and dynamic stretches.
   - Workout:
     - Push-Ups: 3 sets of 12 reps
     - Squats: 3 sets of 15 reps
     - Plank: 3 sets of 30 seconds
     - Lunges: 3 sets of 12 reps per leg
   - **Cool Down (5 minutes):** Stretching major muscle groups.
2. Wednesday: Cardio and Core (25 minutes)
   - **Warm-Up (5 minutes):** Marching in place, arm circles, and leg swings.
   - Workout:
     - Burpees: 3 sets of 10 reps
     - Mountain Climbers: 3 sets of 20 seconds
     - Bicycle Crunches: 3 sets of 15 reps per side
     - Russian Twists: 3 sets of 20 reps
   - **Cool Down (5 minutes):** Yoga poses for core relaxation.
3. Friday: Flexibility and Balance (20 minutes)

- o **Warm-Up (5 minutes):** Gentle jogging in place, side lunges, and hip circles.
- o Workout:
  - ▪ Yoga Flow: Sun salutations, warrior poses, and balance poses like tree pose.
  - ▪ Pilates: Roll-ups, leg circles, and teaser pose.
- o **Cool Down (5 minutes):** Deep breathing and stretching.

Tips to Stay Motivated and Reminded:

1. Set Reminders:
   - o Use your phone or smartwatch to set reminders for your exercise sessions. Apps like MyFitnessPal and Strava have notification features to keep you on track.
2. Visual Cues:
   - o Place workout equipment like resistance bands or dumbbells in visible areas around your home to remind you to use them.
3. Goal Setting:
   - o Set daily or weekly fitness goals. Track your progress using fitness apps. Seeing your achievements can be a great motivator.

4. Social Accountability:
    - Share your fitness goals with friends or join an online fitness community. Social platforms within apps like Strava can help you stay accountable.
5. Rewards:
    - Treat yourself when you hit a fitness milestone. It could be something small like a favorite snack or a new workout outfit.
6. Incorporate Variety:
    - Change your workouts regularly to keep things interesting. Try different exercises or fitness classes to stay engaged.

By embracing home workouts and utilizing bodyweight exercises, you can maintain a consistent fitness routine regardless of your access to a gym. These strategies not only make fitness more accessible but also transform your home into a versatile workout space, making it easier to stay committed and motivated.

Chapter 5: Optimizing Nutrition and Recovery

The Challenge: You and I both know that maintaining a balanced diet and ensuring adequate recovery can be challenging, especially with a busy lifestyle. Poor nutrition and insufficient recovery can significantly hinder your fitness progress and overall health.

The Strategy: Implementing balanced diet plans and effective recovery techniques is crucial. These practices can enhance your energy levels, improve workout performance, and support overall well-being.

Let's Chat: Nutrition and recovery are just as important as your workouts. With your busy schedule, meal prepping can be a game-changer. Preparing balanced meals that are easy to grab and go ensures you're fueling your body properly. Don't forget the importance of recovery—adequate sleep, hydration, and stress management are crucial. These elements help you perform better and feel more energized. Studies have shown that proper nutrition and rest significantly enhance workout performance and overall health.

Key Stats and Insights:

- **Statista Insight:** 45% of professionals admit to having poor eating habits due to their busy schedules, negatively impacting their fitness goals.
- **Expert Quote:** "What you eat and how you recover are just as crucial as your workouts. Proper nutrition and rest can elevate your fitness journey to new heights." – Jessica Shee from iBoysoft.

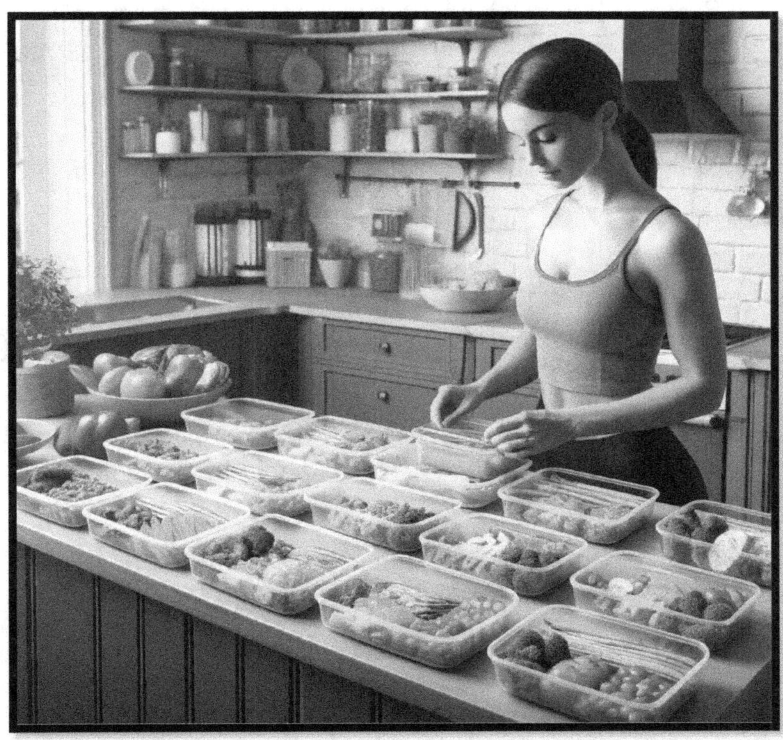

Meal prepping ensures you have healthy meals ready to go.

Paint a Picture:

Imagine this: It's Sunday afternoon, and you've decided to take control of your nutrition for the week. You set up your kitchen and prepare a variety of healthy meals. You chop vegetables, cook quinoa, grill chicken, and assemble mason jar salads. By the end of the afternoon, you have a fridge stocked with balanced, colorful meals. Each day, you grab a prepped meal, knowing it's nutritious and convenient. In the evenings, you ensure you get enough sleep and stay hydrated throughout the day. By the end of the week, you feel more energetic and your workouts have improved significantly.

Why It Works:

- **Convenience:** Meal prepping saves time during the week, making it easier to stick to a healthy diet.
- **Balanced Nutrition:** Prepping meals ensures you get a balanced intake of proteins, carbohydrates, and fats.
- **Recovery:** Proper sleep, hydration, and stress management enhance recovery, allowing your body to repair and strengthen.

Specific Meal Prep Ideas:

Balanced, Colorful Meal Prep Ideas:

1. Rainbow Veggie Bowls:
   - **Ingredients:** Quinoa, chickpeas, cherry tomatoes, bell peppers, red cabbage, spinach, and avocado.
   - **Instructions:** Cook quinoa and chickpeas. Chop vegetables and arrange them in a bowl. Drizzle with a light vinaigrette.
   - Visual:

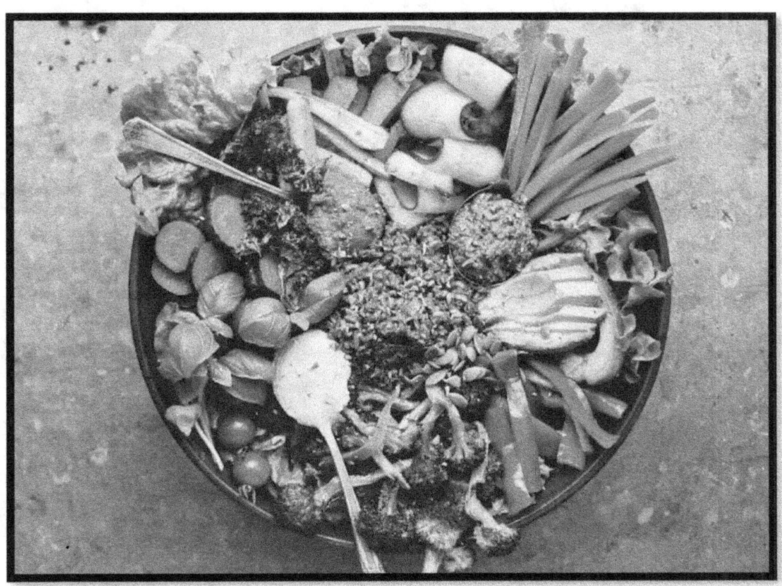

A colorful and nutritious veggie bowl, perfect for meal prepping.

2. Grilled Chicken with Roasted Vegetables:

- o **Ingredients:** Chicken breast, zucchini, carrots, bell peppers, and sweet potatoes.
- o **Instructions:** Grill the chicken and roast the vegetables. Divide into meal prep containers.
- o Visual:

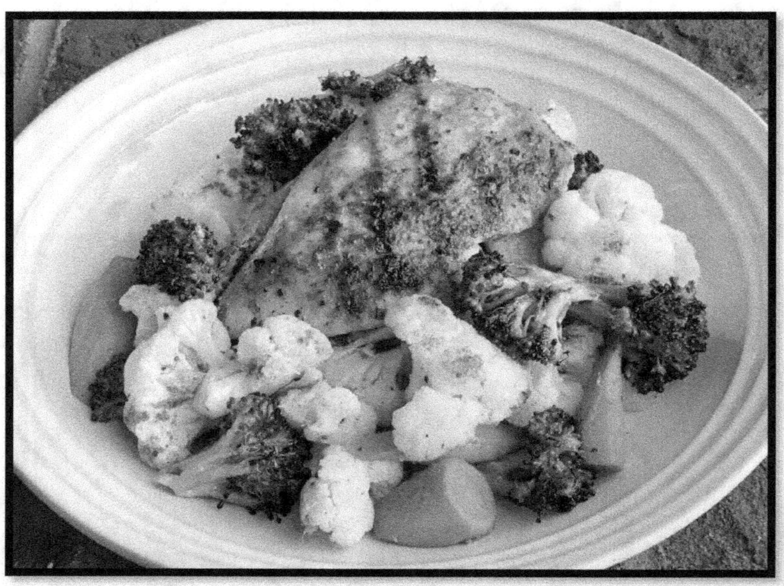

Grilled chicken paired with a medley of roasted vegetables for a balanced meal.

3. Mason Jar Salads:
   - o **Ingredients:** Mixed greens, cherry tomatoes, cucumbers, red onion, olives, feta cheese, and vinaigrette.
   - o **Instructions:** Layer ingredients in a mason jar with the dressing at the

bottom and greens on top. Shake
and eat when ready.
- o Visual:

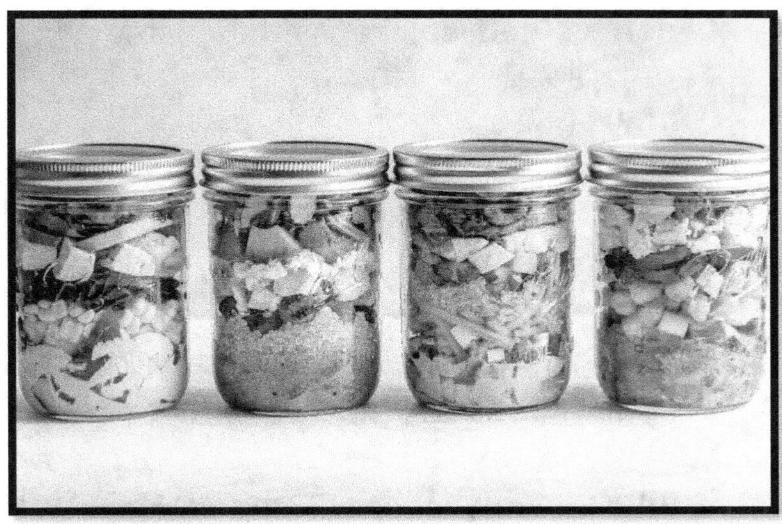

*Mason jar salads are convenient and keep
ingredients fresh.*

Weekly Meal Plan Including Packed Lunches:

Monday:

- **Breakfast:** Greek yogurt with honey and mixed berries.
- **Lunch:** Rainbow Veggie Bowl.
- **Dinner:** Baked salmon with steamed broccoli and brown rice.
- **Snacks:** Apple slices with almond butter, carrot sticks with hummus.

Tuesday:

- **Breakfast:** Overnight oats with chia seeds, almond milk, and sliced bananas.
- **Lunch:** Grilled Chicken with Roasted Vegetables.
- **Dinner:** Stir-fried tofu with mixed vegetables and quinoa.
- **Snacks:** Handful of mixed nuts, Greek yogurt.

Wednesday:

- **Breakfast:** Smoothie with spinach, banana, almond milk, and protein powder.
- **Lunch:** Mason Jar Salad.
- **Dinner:** Turkey chili with black beans and corn.
- **Snacks:** Sliced cucumber with guacamole, boiled eggs.

Thursday:

- **Breakfast:** Scrambled eggs with spinach and whole-grain toast.
- **Lunch:** Rainbow Veggie Bowl.
- **Dinner:** Whole wheat pasta with marinara sauce and grilled chicken.
- **Snacks:** Fresh fruit salad, cheese sticks.

Friday:

- **Breakfast:** Avocado toast with a poached egg.

- **Lunch:** Grilled Chicken with Roasted Vegetables.
- **Dinner:** Baked tilapia with asparagus and quinoa.
- **Snacks:** Smoothie with kale, pineapple, and coconut water, mixed berries.

Saturday:

- **Breakfast:** Whole-grain pancakes with maple syrup and blueberries.
- **Lunch:** Mason Jar Salad.
- **Dinner:** Vegetable stir-fry with tofu and brown rice.
- **Snacks:** Apple slices with peanut butter, yogurt with granola.

Sunday:

- **Breakfast:** Frittata with bell peppers, onions, and mushrooms.
- **Lunch:** Leftover vegetable stir-fry with tofu.
- **Dinner:** Roast chicken with sweet potatoes and green beans.
- **Snacks:** Orange slices, trail mix.

Tips to Stay Motivated and Reminded:

1. Set Reminders:
   - Use your phone or smartwatch to set reminders for your exercise sessions. Apps like MyFitnessPal and Strava

have notification features to keep you on track.

2. Visual Cues:
   o Place workout equipment like resistance bands or dumbbells in visible areas around your home to remind you to use them.
3. Goal Setting:
   o Set daily or weekly fitness goals. Track your progress using fitness apps. Seeing your achievements can be a great motivator.
4. Social Accountability:
   o Share your fitness goals with friends or join an online fitness community. Social platforms within apps like Strava can help you stay accountable.
5. Rewards:
   o Treat yourself when you hit a fitness milestone. It could be something small like a favorite snack or a new workout outfit.
6. Incorporate Variety:
   o Change your workouts regularly to keep things interesting. Try different exercises or fitness classes to stay engaged.

Convenience Tips:

1. Prepare Meals in Bulk:
    - Cooking in bulk saves time and ensures you have healthy meals ready throughout the week. For example, cook a large batch of quinoa or grill several chicken breasts at once.
2. Use Quality Storage Containers:
    - Invest in high-quality, leak-proof containers to keep your meals fresh. Look for BPA-free options that are microwave and dishwasher safe.
    - Recommended Containers:
        - Glass Meal Prep Containers:
            - Glass Meal Prep Containers on Amazon
        - Bento Lunch Box Containers:
            - Bento Lunch Box Containers on Amazon
        - Mason Jars for Salads:
            - Mason Jars on Amazon

By focusing on balanced nutrition and proper recovery techniques, you can significantly enhance your fitness journey. These strategies not only improve your performance but also ensure you stay healthy and energized, making it easier to maintain a consistent and effective fitness routine.

Conclusion

Recap What You've Learned

We've tackled the top five challenges that busy professionals face in maintaining their fitness:

1. **Time Constraints:** Implementing quick, efficient workout routines like HIIT that can fit into any schedule.
2. **Lack of Motivation:** Using achievable goals, tracking progress with fitness apps, and finding community support to stay motivated.
3. **Difficulty Maintaining Consistency:** Adopting flexible fitness plans that integrate exercise into daily activities, no matter how unpredictable your schedule.
4. **Lack of Accessible Resources:** Utilizing home workouts and bodyweight exercises that require minimal to no equipment, transforming any space into a personal gym.
5. **Nutrition and Recovery:** Preparing balanced meals through meal prepping and emphasizing the importance of adequate recovery, including sleep and hydration.

Call to Action

Ready to transform your fitness journey? Start today by integrating these strategies into your routine and experience the benefits of a healthier, more energized life. Embrace these changes and unlock your full potential, no matter how busy your schedule is.

Nuggets and Tips to Stay Fit

1. Visual Aids for Progress:
    - Keep visual records of your fitness progress. Use photos, measurements, or progress charts to stay motivated and see your improvements over time.
2. Infographics:
    - **Benefits of HIIT:** Create an infographic summarizing the benefits of HIIT. This can help you quickly understand and communicate the advantages of high-intensity workouts.
    - **Quick Desk Exercises:** Develop a visual guide for quick desk exercises. This ensures you can stay active even during long work hours.
    - **Meal Prep Timeline:** Design a meal prep timeline showing how to plan

weekly meals efficiently. This makes meal prepping straightforward and ensures you have nutritious meals ready to go.

Where to Find These Templates:

- **Benefits of HIIT Infographic:** You can download customizable templates from sites like Canva.
- **Quick Desk Exercises Visual Guide:** Find templates on Visme.
- **Meal Prep Timeline Template:** Get detailed and editable templates from Piktochart.

Additional Tips:

1. Set Reminders:
   - Use your phone or smartwatch to set reminders for your exercise sessions. Apps like MyFitnessPal and Strava have notification features to keep you on track.
2. Visual Cues:
   - Place workout equipment like resistance bands or dumbbells in visible areas around your home to remind you to use them.
3. Goal Setting:
   - Set daily or weekly fitness goals. Track your progress using fitness

apps. Seeing your achievements can be a great motivator.

4. Social Accountability:
   - Share your fitness goals with friends or join an online fitness community. Social platforms within apps like Strava can help you stay accountable.
5. Rewards:
   - Treat yourself when you hit a fitness milestone. It could be something small like a favorite snack or a new workout outfit.
6. Incorporate Variety:
   - Change your workouts regularly to keep things interesting. Try different exercises or fitness classes to stay engaged.

By focusing on balanced nutrition and proper recovery techniques, you can significantly enhance your fitness journey. These strategies not only improve your performance but also ensure you stay healthy and energized, making it easier to maintain a consistent and effective fitness routine.

References:

1. Statista - Fitness Insights
2. Healthline - Benefits of HIIT

About the Author

Fit Gal will transform your life by integrating fitness seamlessly into your hectic schedules.

Contact me at <u>mrynne7@hotmail.com</u>

Stay connected for more fitness tips, personalized plans, and exclusive offers. Join our mailing list and receive a free meal prep guide to kickstart your fitness journey!